What people s‌a

GW01315728

"This book changed me

Being a real exercise and workout fanatic, I began to suffer from stiffness in my lower back and hamstrings and was told to have a rest from exercise for 3-4 weeks. Unfortunately, resting seemed to make it worse, which I found very frustrating as I was so used to being active and fit.

I knew Colin from the local fitness center and I explained to him one day why I had been absent for a few weeks and he advised me to start doing some specific stretching exercises, Rag Doll (my favorite)... and I started doing these stretches twice a day and within a few days noticed a real improvement.

I was soon back exercising again, but this time I included these stretches in my cool down and have since kept any stiffness at bay. A great result for me."

– *Louise Martin*

"I first met Colin as a complete stranger at the finish of a hilly 14 mile run Race Event.

We were in a small group comparing our run times and medals when I mentioned that I had an annoying backache and lower back pain.

He shortly took me to one side and showed me two specific exercises which he suggested be done at home. The first I remember he called Rag Doll and the second he named the Cobra, both of which he mentions in his new book. I now practice both exercises, along with others, at least three times a week *and*, since then, no more back problems. Thanks Colin."

– *Lee Mitchell*

Praise for *The Back Pain Survival Guide*

"*The Back Pain Survival Guide* is a truly amazing book documenting the author's unique expertise and experience on the subject of acute back pain.

The illustrations and explanations are easily understood and provide self-explanatory methods for self-help.

The Cobra exercise and illustrations in particular have been particularly useful in helping me back to a normal pain free life.

I later discovered that the Cobra position is a well known Yoga position for the back and helps the back to move in all directions by keeping it supple.

I practice the Cobra exercise on a daily basis for just a few minutes and I have had no recurrence of my problem."

— *Helen Tate*

"This book changed my life. I had suffered 'sciatica' on and off for several years without finding a complete positive solution, until I was recommended *The Back Pain Survival Guide.*

In my particular case, my sciatica always occurred on my right side and was quickly eased with one special exercise which I followed to bring quick relief from my pain.

There are many comprehensive illustrations in this book which I liked because they can be easily followed."

— *Cory Hartley*

THE BACK PAIN SURVIVAL GUIDE

7 Simple Steps to a Pain-Free Back

Colin Platt

First Printing: 2021

Copyright © 2021 by Colin Platt

All rights reserved.

This book or any of its parts may not be reproduced or used in any manner whatsoever without the express written permission of the author and publisher. However, brief quotations in a book review or scholarly journal are permitted.

This book is not intended to be medical advice. The information contained in this book is for educational purposes only and no responsibility will be accepted by the author or publisher for any actions taken related to such information.

Any attempt to diagnose and treat any condition should be done under the direction of a healthcare professional.

Because each person and situation is unique, the author and publisher urge the reader to carefully select the appropriate qualified health professional or other healthcare providers.

The author is not associated with any product described or mentioned in this book.

Contents

1 Introduction 13

    Meeting the Therapist *16*

    A Quick Note on Breathing *18*

2 The Exercises..19

    Posture *20*

    Rag Doll *22*

    The Bridge *24*

    Side Bend..*26*

    The Huggie...*28*

    The Cat Camel...*30*

    Back Stretch..*32*

    The Cobra Extension *34*

3 Pregnancy and Core Training-Prenatal
Pelvic Floor Exercises..37

    First trimester (0-12 weeks) *38*

    Second trimester (13-26 weeks)................................*40*

    Third trimester (27-40 weeks) *42*

4 Conquer Your Core 45

    The Benefits of Core Training *47*

    Push-ups *48*

    Can't Do Push-ups?..*50*

5 Additional Exercises 51

	Stretching	52
	Shoulder Stretches	54
	Wall Push Ups	56
6	Pain Avoidance Tips	59
	Lifting Correctly	60
	Deportment	62
	The Posture Corrector	64
7	Viewing The Anatomy	67
	Shoulder Joint	68
	The Sciatic Nerve	70
8	Therapists to Help Back Pain	73
	Physical Therapists (PT)	74
	Chiropractors (DC)	75
	Osteopaths	76
	Acupuncture	77
9	Reflexology	79
10	Working From Home	81
11	Keeping Going	85
12	Also Written by Colin Platt	87
13	Physical Therapy Association Offices	91
14	Index	99

Free Gift!

As a "thank-you" for getting this book, I'd like to give you a free gift: a unique PDF called: *Indoor and Outdoor Aerobic Exercises for Cold Weather.*

Here is the link: www.backpainsolved.com/inout

Enjoy!

Acknowledgements

I want to thank all the people who have helped me in writing this book.

To family and friends and to my wife Judy in particular who made sure that there was food on the table at regular intervals during my writing regime!

With thanks to Pippa my daughter with her qualified rehabilitation skills and exercise plans, and to Tony my son for his enthusiastic support and for never doubting my ability to see my project to its final stage.

Tony Crofts for the editing, his technical assistance, and general advice. Contact Tony at: *tonymicroft@gmail.com*

Finally, many thanks to Chris Payne for his unwavering support and advice with the structure of this book. Without his help, this book would have been a non-starter. *www.christopherjohnpayne.com*

About the Author

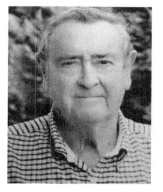

A number of years ago Colin used to be in constant pain. It took over his life and he could hardly think about anything else. Now he is pain free. He did this by taking advice from physicians, chiropractors and physical therapists to create a simple exercise plan that he followed every day. Within a few days he was free from pain.

Now in his 80s, he attributes his vibrant health to following this simple roadmap.

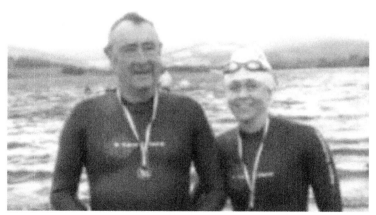

Taken after a 1-mile charity swim with his daughter Pippa in 2013 when he was 75 years young!

Chapter 1

Introduction

Anyone who has ever suffered back pain knows that the pain can be excruciating and seriously, seriously painful.

In my case, it happened when I was least expecting it at about 14 miles into one of my marathon training runs when I tripped over my dog. Sorry, Tess.

I was obviously not alone! Tess my faithful dog, a small border collie cross, was ambling just ahead and to one side of me.

I guess I was tiring without realizing, tripped, and stumbled over a black and white furry thing; I managed to save myself from falling, in doing so I felt a twinge in my lower back.

I realized it would be foolish to carry on as I knew physically that my run was over for the day, as well as my faithful companions. To carry on would make matters worse.

Limping home slowly with Tess in my arms was my only option. I was more worried about Tess than myself, but she did lick my face as we pottered home.

I had pain in the back of my right leg and by now and it had traveled from my buttock to my right foot, which was now tingling.

Later that day, I tried hot and cold packs on my lower back and found some relief but I realized that this was not the immediate answer. In the meantime, my daughter arrived home from her gym and she quickly took charge.

"Tess is ok" she said. "Just bruised, but I am more concerned about you at this stage."

Being a certified level 3 personal fitness trainer, she was able to diagnose Sciatica immediately. Insisting, before anything else, that I carry out some very gentle stretching which she called **Rag Doll**.

The sequence of Rag Doll is demonstrated and detailed in the exercise section on page 22.

"In the meantime," she said, "painkillers like ibuprofen or paracetamol may help and I should take them regularly at the recommended doses if I needed them."

Note: For the ladies, aspirin, and ibuprofen should *not* be taken if you are pregnant, if in doubt you should check with your pharmacist.

The Back Pain Survival Guide

Meeting the Therapist

To continue with my story… I persevered with the Rag Doll exercise over the next 48 hours together with the Huggie exercise (page 28) which I found particularly helpful to relieve my back pain. So much so that I decided to try to make my way to my Gym and rehab center the following morning for some more essential advice from an expert physical therapist.

The pain had now moved to my lower back, which the therapist said was a common source of pain for some athletes.

As the therapist worked on my back, he explained that my discomfort was likely due to my gait, height and, in particular, my posture. He talked about posture and carriage explaining that in my case some specific abdominal exercises were an essential part of my rehabilitation… when I was able!

He worked on my back for nearly an hour, talking as he worked, asking me to return the following day, if possible, to check out my posture. I was very fortunate to have a physical therapist available at such short notice, an expert in musculoskeletal problems.

He explained that posture deformities are even more pronounced in the elderly and can become a habit if not recognized early. As posture is so important when doing all the exercises, I'll talk about that next and then go on to show you what the exercises are and tell you how to do them. In some of the exercise steps, I've added some fine detail to help.

The Back Pain Survival Guide

A Quick Note on Breathing

Breath control is also a significant part of these gentle exercise routines.

Remember to always only breathe through your nose and *not* through your mouth.

I know this is probably different from what most instructors say but here's why…

Your nose is connected to your sinuses which filter incoming air. Saves you from sucking in a lot of the rubbish that is in the air, even if we can't actually see it.

Your nasal passages need to be kept moist in order to work properly. Breathing out through your nose achieves this.

If you breathe out through your mouth, after just a few breaths your nasal passages will dry and not work properly. This will become uncomfortable, so it is an automatic reaction to breathe through your mouth instead.

Over time, mouth breathing becomes a habit that encourages a host of ailments which you'll probably never attribute to being because of the way you breathe. Asthma being the prime example

You also get up to 25% more Oxygen by breathing both in and out through your nose.

Now let's get on to posture and the exercises.

Chapter 2

The Exercises

Posture

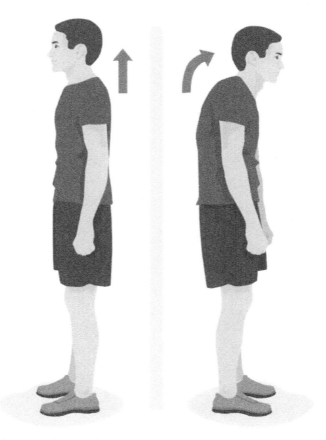

Look carefully at the above image.

Slouching or stooping can very easily become a habit over time because it causes overstretching of the ligaments in the shoulders.

The Exercises

Posture

The main cause of habitual stooping can be caused as follows:

- Sitting for a long time in the same position, such as watching TV.

- Playing computer games.

- A computer monitor or laptop at the incorrect height.

- Bending over in the incorrect position whilst gardening.

- Pushing a wheelbarrow.

- Lifting heavy objects incorrectly

- Poor standing and lying postures.

Correct posture is a good habit,
not just an exercise.
A habit to be practiced every day!

Rag Doll

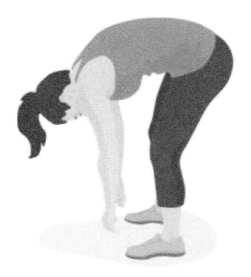

The important thing to remember with this exercise is **not to bounce**.

The exercise should be carried out with a very controlled motion that will gently stretch the muscles in the lower back and the hamstrings tendons at the back of the legs.

The Exercises

Rag Doll

- Stand with feet shoulder-width apart, a straight back, and soft knees, pull your tummy in to engage your abdominal core muscles at the same time squeeze your butt cheeks together

  IMPORTANT: This is called 'engaging your core.'

- Inhale gently through your nose then slowly exhale, also through your nose.

- Tucking in your chin and *keeping your* shoulders, *head, and neck relaxed,* roll forward in a smooth controlled motion. *Suck in your belly button, but do not hold your breath.*

- With your arms hanging loose and elbows relaxed, slowly roll down as if going to touch your toes.

- Continue this movement until you are fully folded.

- Hold for a few breaths and then *slowly* roll back up and return to the standing position.

- Repeat two or three times until you are feeling quite relaxed.

The Bridge

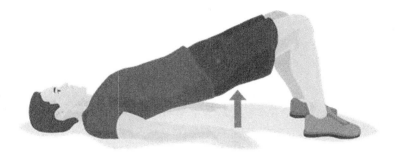

This simple but effective exercise is important as it helps to improve posture – especially when you spend a lot of your time at home sitting at your desk.

It activates the muscles in your lower back and assists your abdominal midsection.

- Lie on your back with your knees bent and your feet flat on the floor just hip-width apart, arms and hands as shown.

The Exercises

The Bridge

- Exhale.

- Engage your core and slowly raise your hips as high off the floor as possible and clench your butt cheeks. (Glutes).

  Note, keep the weight on your shoulders and off your neck.

- Hold this position for 5 breaths at the top of the movement then slowly, with control, sink to the floor.

- Repeat three times, twice or three times daily.

  A more advanced position to this exercise would be to exhale and place your hands under your rib cage to support the posture and lift your trunk higher, parallel with the ceiling.

- Breathe steadily for 5 breaths then slowly return to your starting position.

The Back Pain Survival Guide

Side Bend

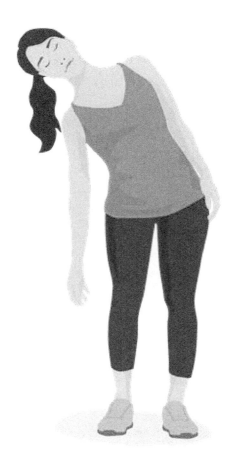

The Exercises

Side Bend

This simple exercise is an effective way to stretch your side muscles (Obliques) to stabilize your spine.

- Stand with your feet shoulder-width apart straight back and soft knees.

- Keeping your head in line with your spine, bend from the waist towards your knee.

- Return to the start, then repeat to the other side.

The Back Pain Survival Guide

The Huggie

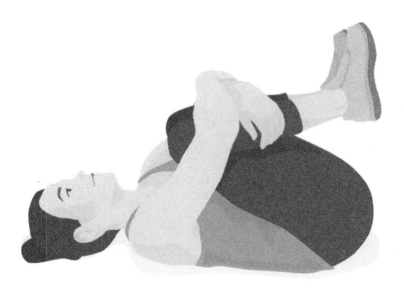

The Exercises

The Huggie

The Huggie is the ideal exercise to ease the pain of sciatic nerve pain and assist rehabilitation. A small flat cushion or book behind the head is recommended.

The Huggie is very similar to the crunch but involves bringing your legs closer to the body. It works the lower abdominals with less stress on your neck and shoulders.

- Lie on your back with bent knees and feet flat on the floor.

- Bend one knee and with your hands pull it in to your chest trailing the other leg.

- Do the same with the other leg. Finally pull both knees towards the stomach.

- Hug your legs as shown into the body and very gently rock gently side-to-side to massage your lower back.

- Hold this position for 5 breaths and repeat 3 times.

The Cat Camel

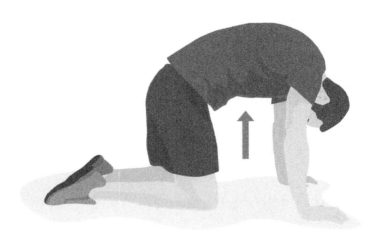

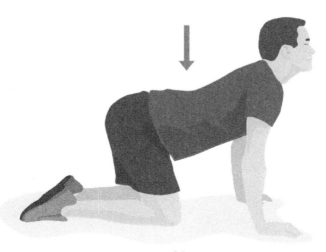

The Exercises

The Cat Camel

The purpose of this exercise is to reduce back stiffness. It also helps to lubricate the spine and increase your flexibility.

This is a great exercise and can be done as part of your warm-up routine.

- Begin on all fours with your hands flat on the floor in line with your shoulders and knees below your hips.

- Inhale and slowly lower your head, pull your stomach in at the same time as raising your back.

- Exhale and hold this position for about 5 seconds at the top of the movement, feeling the stretch in your back.

- In one movement, arch your back whilst looking straight ahead. Hold this position for another 5 seconds then return to normal.

- This exercise can be done several times until you feel comfortable and relaxed.

Back Stretch

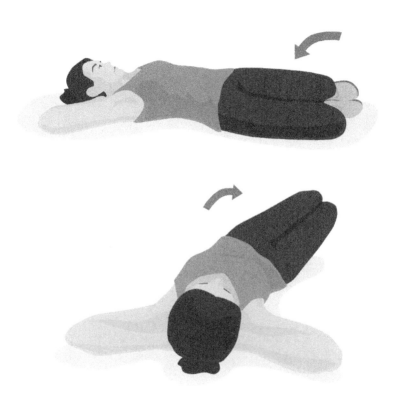

This exercise strengthens the lower back, exercises the abdominal muscles and, at the same time, improves and stretches the mid and lower back. All essential areas you need to maintain to keep your back healthy and pain free.

The Exercises

Back Stretch

- To start, place your hands behind your head to help brace the body against the floor. *This to prevents the body from rolling from side to side and assists in keeping the shoulders in a stable position.* Keep your feet on the floor.

- Keep your shoulders flat to the floor; engage your core.

- With knees together, raise your legs 90 degrees while keeping your lower back stable.

- Still keeping your shoulders flat on the floor, tense your core muscles to control the next movement.

- Slowly roll your hips and legs to the **right** and hold this position for 5 breaths.

- In the same manner, engage your core and slowly roll to the **left,** hold for 5 breaths.

- Repeat as many times as feels comfortable.

The Cobra Extension

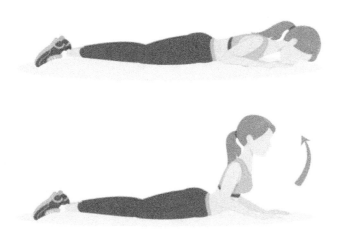

The simple exercise is designed to strengthen the lower back muscles and improve spinal flexibility.

If your back is sore it will easier for you to practice this whilst standing.

This is also a well-known yoga extension posture for keeping your back and body supple and is designed to strengthen the lower back muscles and improve your spinal flexibility.

The Exercises

The Cobra Extension

The Cobra is now my favorite exercise and I recommend this exercise for you to do in bed *every morning* as a starter for an exercise regime to keep your back strong and supple.

The Cobra Extension in the prone position

- Lie face down with your hands flat on the floor level with your chin, as shown.

- Exhale and push up with your arms to lift your head and shoulders off the floor. *Raise your head and shoulders as high as comfortable — do not lift your hips as this prevents the arch.*

- Hold this position for 5 breaths and then release down. *(This exercise can easily be practiced in bed before you get up in the morning.)*

The Back Pain Survival Guide

The Cobra Extension in the standing position

- Start by placing your hands in the small of your back with fingertips facing downwards.

- Bend backwards and hold the position for 5 deep breaths.

- This exercise should be repeated five times as a set.

- Repeat several times daily.

Chapter 3

Pregnancy and Core Training-Prenatal Pelvic Floor Exercises

First trimester (0-12 weeks)

Toe Tap

It is essential to build and maintain a strong core during pregnancy. This is vital to avoid back pain, hip pain, and sciatica

It is imperative start these pelvic floor-core exercises as soon as possible.

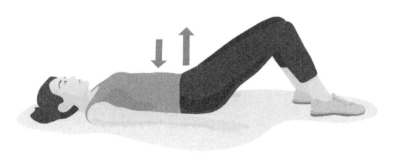

Pelvic floor exercises are vitally important in pregnancy and it is essential to start activating them as soon as possible.

Pregnancy and Core Training

First trimester (0-12 weeks)

Toe Tap

This is a core stabilizing exercise strengthens the muscles of your abdomen which may lead to reduced back pain.

- Keeping your core engaged, lift your right leg so that your hip and knee are at right angles while keeping your left foot on the floor.

- Lift your left leg until it is level with the right.

- Hold this position for a few seconds, then return to the starting position.

- Still keeping your core engaged, repeat but reverse the order of the leg lifts

To progress, try the more demanding exercise by lifting both legs at once so that both hip and knees are at right angles, hold for a few seconds and lower your feet to the floor.

It is important to engage your core engaged, and to breathe normally throughout.

Second trimester (13-26 weeks)

The Prenatal Bridge

This exercise helps to reduce back pain in the second trimester of pregnancy by activating and strengthening the muscles in the pelvis and lower back.

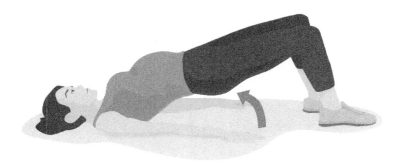

Pregnancy and Core Training

Second trimester (13-26 weeks)

- Lie on your back with your knees bent and your feet flat on the floor just hip-width apart, arms and hands as shown.

- Exhale: engage your core and slowly raise your hips as high off the floor as possible and clench your butt cheeks. (Glutes).

- Inhale; keep the weight on your shoulders and off your neck. Hold this position for five breaths at the top of the movement.

- Slowly, with control, lower to the floor.

- Repeat three times, two or three times daily.

Third trimester (27-40 weeks)

Core Training and strengthening to helping to prepare for baby delivery.

Prenatal: Superwoman

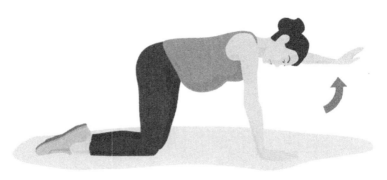

Core Training and strengthening, helping to prepare for delivery.

This exercise strengthens your pelvic floor and improves core balance and builds stability and strength in your lower back, and shoulders.

Starting on all fours, with your knees at right angles to your hips, and your hands under the shoulders pointing forwards and the back straight.

This will help your baby into the correct position.

Third trimester (27-40 weeks)

From this starting position, engage your core and at the same raise one arm in front of you. Hold for 5 breaths and return to the start position and now raise the other arm similarly.

To progress

When you feel at ease with the first exercise, assume the start position with your core engaged and this time with one straight leg raised out horizontally behind you at hip height. This will demand deep core control and balance.

As previously, hold for 5 breaths, return and raise the opposite arm.

To progress further to Superwoman

When you feel at ease and with one arm raised, as in the image, again from the start position with your core engaged raise the opposite leg horizontally and hold for 5 breaths, return and raise the opposite arm and opposite leg maintaining a straight line throughout from your shoulders to your hips.

Chapter 4

Conquer Your Core

The Back Pain Survival Guide

In recent years, there has been much talk about the importance of a strong core. There is a proven reason for this. The core is where much of the powerful movements of the body initiate, so really it might be called your "Power Center."

When people hear about the "core," they automatically think of the abdominals. However, the core is more complex than having a great "six-pack." The core consists of different muscles that work together to support the upper and lower body.

The secret to success with core strength training is to stabilize, or tense, your core before and during each exercise.

Stabilizing the core can be described as, 'tensing the core,' 'engaging the core,' 'activating the core,' 'tightening the core,' 'contracting the core.' Whatever it is called, it all means the same in every case. Maintaining a 'tensed' core during each and every exercise, as well as tightening the 'Glutes' i.e. your buttocks.

To 'tense' the core, simply contract your belly button towards your spine remembering not to hold your breath. Just breathe normally.

Engaging your core will help to stabilize your body, making sure it is in the correct alignment for your workout.

Now be aware of your posture. Do not slouch. Start the exercises below to fire up your core and build a rock-solid body.

Note: The Bridge exercise on page 24 is the ideal 'starters' exercise to begin your core strength training.

> *Correct posture is a good habit,*
> *not just an exercise.*
> *A habit to be practiced every day!*

The Benefits of Core Training

- Back pain reduced or eliminated
- Better posture prevents 'slouching'
- Improved balance
- Reduced risk of back injury
- Increased athletic performance
- More efficient transfer of energy
- An increased sense of health, power and ability

When your shoulder and back pain has improved, and you have *consulted your physician and or your physical trainer*, you might like to start some simple core strength exercises.

The Back Pain Survival Guide

Push-ups

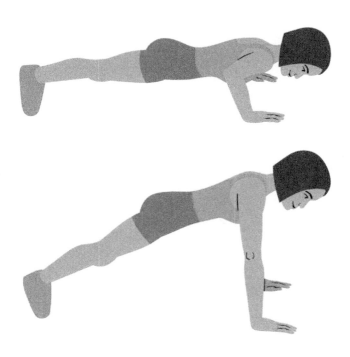

Push ups

To complete a perfect push-up:

- Start in the prone position with your hands level with your shoulders.

- Engage your core.

- Raise your body by pressing into the floor, keeping your body horizontal.

- Lower and repeat for as many times as you feel comfortable.

Note for beginners
You will find this core push-up exercise easier by completing a few sets balancing on your knees instead of your toes.

Another popular variation of this exercise is to place the hands slightly wider than the shoulders; this will build upper body strength and is an ideal exercise for working the upper back, shoulders, biceps, core and abdominals.

Can't Do Push-ups?

Instead of the Wall Push-ups on page 56, why not try gentle inclined push-ups whilst on a block, a solid chair or a step, as in the image below.

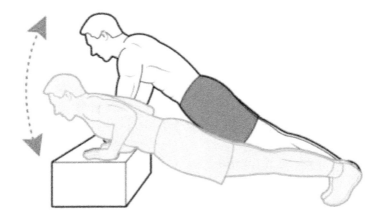

Can't do push-ups?

Here's how to make a start.

- Place the palms a little wider than shoulder width apart on the edge of a table or step.

- Step backwards and lean as the image above.

- Lower your chest as far down as comfortable, and then push back up.

Chapter 5

Additional Exercises

Stretching

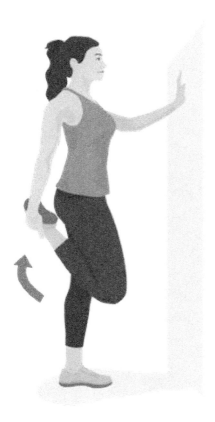

Additional Exercises

Stretching

This standing quadriceps exercise, in the illustration above, will stretch the hip and thigh muscles keeping these muscles flexible. It may also control back and knee pain.

Hold this position as shown for 30 seconds then switch to the left leg.

This is considered the safest way to stretch. Done gently, without bouncing, allows the connective tissue to reset to its original state.

What's the difference between dynamic and static stretching?

Typically, dynamic stretching is done before you begin a workout and involves active progressive movements that help your muscles warm up ready for exercise.

Static stretching is done at the end of an active workout and involves a series of stretches which you hold for about 30 seconds. These exercises increase your range of motion and flexibility.

The Back Pain Survival Guide

Shoulder Stretches

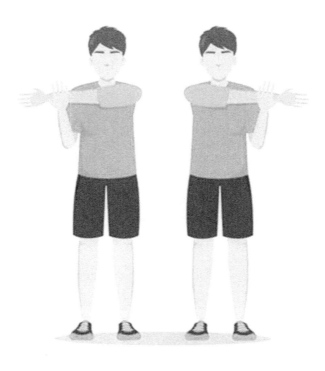

Additional Exercises

Shoulder Stretches

As we age, our range of motion decreases and some movement problems can occur.

Simple shoulder stretching exercises, as above, improve flexibility and range of motion of the shoulder structure.

Try to remember to carry out the above shoulder stretches exercise as part of your warm-up or warm-down routine but try to avoid any painful movements.

Aim for a balance between activity and rest.

If you have prolonged discomfort and your symptoms show no sign of improving after two weeks, please contact your physician.

The Back Pain Survival Guide

Wall Push Ups

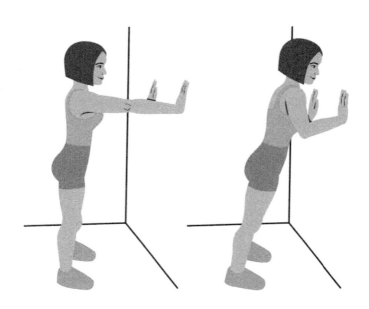

Additional Exercises

Wall Push Ups

Many people with **shoulder pain** struggle to complete even one standard push-up. By that, I mean the horizontal floor exercise.

Therefore, one of the best exercises to help with your shoulder pain is the wall-push up *and,* as a bonus, you will achieve stronger arms, chest muscles, back and abdominals.

My recommendation to master this popular exercise is to start the exercise as a wall push-up as illustrated, before attempting the horizontal version.

To set yourself up for success follow these simple steps.

- Place your palms on the wall, shoulder-distance apart at shoulder height.

- Place your feet at shoulder width.

- Now stand as close to the wall as you feel comfortable to complete ten push-ups.
  During this exercise, it is important to engage (tense) your core muscles (abdominals) and keep the back engaged.

The Back Pain Survival Guide

Wall Push Ups

- Inhale as you bend your elbows.

- Bring your chest closer to the wall, keeping the elbows pointing downwards.

- Exhale as you push gently away and return to the starting position.
  As you become stronger, you should be able to complete three sets of 15 each, three times per week.

For some fun variation, try performing this exercise in a doorway with your hands slightly above your head.

- Slowly lean forward until you are stretching the front of your shoulders.

- Hold for 10-20 seconds, then push back again.

- Repeat three times.

  To make this exercise more of a challenge when you are able, gradually move your feet further from the wall.

  The secret is to have fun completing these exercises.

Chapter 6

Pain Avoidance Tips

The Back Pain Survival Guide

Lifting Correctly

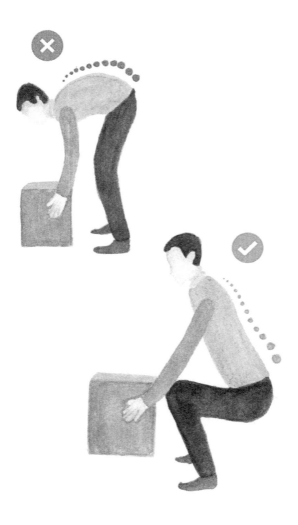

Lifting Correctly

The left-hand image is **totally incorrect**. Notice the curved spine and straight legs… a recipe for a bad back!

To minimize damage to your back, always stand close to the object to be lifted as in the right-hand image above. Bending your knees to keep your back straight.

- Hinge from your hips using your strong thigh muscles (quadriceps).

- Stand close to the load with your feet hip width apart.

- Bend your knees keeping your back straight.

- With a straight back lift steadily, do not jerk.

- When lowering a load, use the same technique.

Deportment

Correct posture allows people from around the world to carry heavy loads all day without causing back pain.

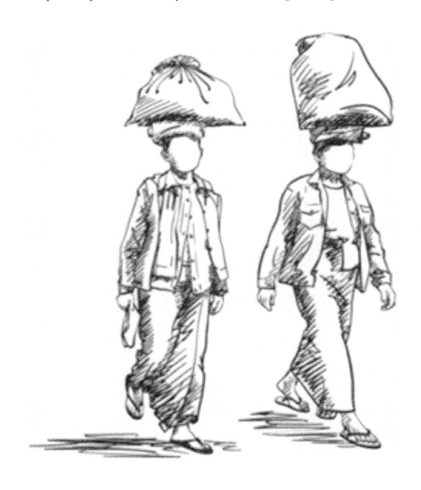

Deportment

Just look carefully at the facing image. Many people in the developing world are known to balance and carry loads of up to 75% of their own body weight on their heads. How do they manage this remarkable feat?

Much of what I have learnt over the years has always emphasized the importance of body posture and deportment to help with avoiding or easing back pain.

You would imagine the enormous loading to their spine and spinal discs would damage their spines, causing major back pain. On the contrary. Without realizing, they are using their anterior core muscles. They are the ones to the side of the abdomen working with those of the back and buttocks acting like a corset, thus stabilizing the spine. Amazingly, when the head is loaded with such a weight, the neck muscles and spine act in a vertical way to support it!

The Posture Corrector

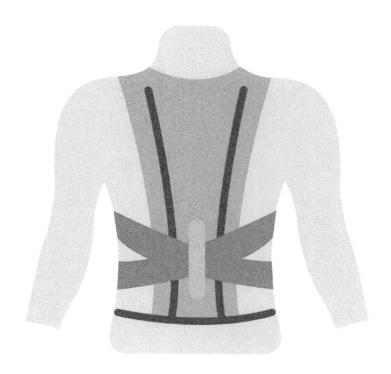

Image viewed from the back

Posture braces are the perfect answer for people who spend a lot of time hunched over at work. They bring the shoulders together, improving posture and making wearers aware of poor hunched postures.

The Posture Corrector

Braces eliminate back, neck, and shoulder pain to give perfect posture by ensuring the wearer stands taller and is prevented from stooping.

If you have rounded shoulders and have a tendency to slouch, this device will provide gentle correction.

These braces are lightweight, made of fabric and adjustable nylon tape. They are easy to wear under clothing and are available for both men and women.

However, these braces are not a substitute for improving muscle strength in your back through exercise!

Costing between $20 and $30 they are readily available from sporting goods stores, local pharmacies and online.

Chapter 7

Viewing The Anatomy

Shoulder Joint

How the Shoulder Works

The shoulder is a ball and socket arrangement and is the most mobile joint in the whole body,

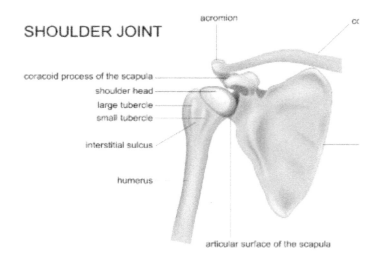

Just a group of four muscles and their tendons make up what is called the *rotator cuff*. This controls movement and also assists to keep the joint mobile while working to keep the head of your upper arm within the shoulder socket.

Viewing The Anatomy

Shoulder Joint

Shoulder pain may be part of a general condition such as osteoarthritis or rheumatoid arthritis, the most common cause of pain over the outside of the shoulder is usually a rotator cuff problem.

Rotator cuff injuries are very common and can increase with age. Such injuries are more common with people who have jobs that require repeatedly performing arm motions such as plasterers (very common), painters, and even hairdressers.

Frozen Shoulder

A common condition that involves stiffness of the joint, discomfort when dressing, and loss of movement when reaching behind.

Sometimes a corticosteroid injection will help, given under X-ray conditions.

Since there are many potential causes of shoulder pain for this complicated shoulder structure it is wise to seek a thorough medical examination as soon as possible, after which you will be referred to a physical therapist.

The Sciatic Nerve

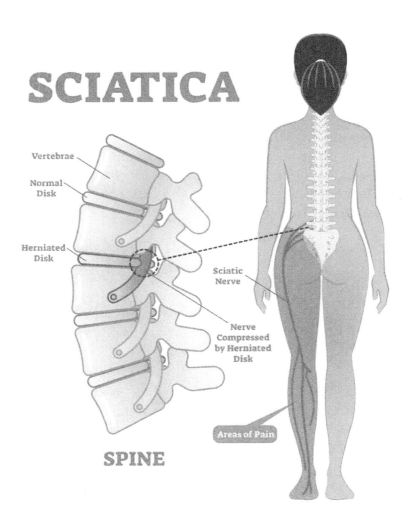

The Sciatic Nerve

These nerves are approximately ¾ inch (2cms) in diameter and are the largest nerves in the body. They start in the lower back and run down the back of each leg. When affected, they can often be associated with tingling, numbness, and weakness in the leg and foot. Typically, sciatica affects only one side of the body.

The back is a complicated structure formed around the bones of the spinal column and is the central axis of the spinal column. This consists of 24 bones (vertebrae) sitting on top of each other.

It sits on the pelvis and goes up to the skull.

The bones of the spine are connected by discs at the front and facet joints at the back.

It is part of the axial skeleton, extending from the base of the skull down to the tip of the coccyx. The bottom bone of the backbone.

The spinal cord runs through the center.

In most cases, pain from a sciatic nerve can be sudden and persist for a number of days. The pain is caused by a number of conditions that lead to the compression of the nerve as it exits the spinal cord.

The Huggie (page 28) is the ideal exercise to ease sciatic nerve pain and assist rehabilitation. A small flat cushion or book behind the head is recommended.

Chapter 8

Therapists to Help Back Pain

Physical therapists or physiotherapists, chiropractors and osteopaths are all qualified professionals who can treat back pain with manual therapies, but they have different treatment techniques.

Physical Therapists (PT)

Physical therapy, or physiotherapy, is the treatment of individuals suffering from injuries or long-term disabilities. Also helping reduce your risk of injury in the future.

At your first appointment, you will have an assessment to determine what help you may need.

They treat conditions such as chronic back pain, soft tissue injuries, cartilage damage, posture and gait disorders.

Chiropractors (DC)

Chiropractors use manual manipulation to align any musculoskeletal issues. Seven million Americans pursue this type of treatment, particularly for the back and spine.

The initials "DC" identify a chiropractor who has attended an undergraduate degree and 4 years at a chiropractic college.

Apart from manipulation, many give advice on nutrition and exercise plans. Most of the exercises making up those plans are detailed in this book for you.

Osteopaths

An osteopath uses physical manipulation and stretching. Most commonly used to treat back pain and other musculoskeletal conditions.

An osteopath will check your posture from the hips upwards, and check that your head is in alignment in your normal posture position.

See page 20.

Acupuncture

Acupuncture began in China more than 2,400 years ago and involves the practice of inserting thin needles at certain 'meridian' points in the body which may help to relieve chronic back pain.

The good news is research shows acupuncture may be an effective tool for treating back pain by stimulating the central nervous system to release chemicals into the spinal cord triggering the release of natural opioids in the brain.

Chapter 9

Reflexology

The Back Pain Survival Guide

Reflexology

Reflexology is a technique that applies gentle pressure to your hands and feet or ears to help relieve tension in the body and to bring about a state of relaxation to aid the healing process and relieve pain.

It works in a similar manner to acupuncture, and the theory of the process involves particular points in the body that correspond to certain reflex areas and organs in the body.

By applying pressure to these areas a reflexologist is said to remove blockages and promote health to a designated area.

Your physician would initially advise which expert to consult for your particular condition.

Chapter 10

Working From Home

The Back Pain Survival Guide

A physical therapist can give you invaluable advice to ease back pain situation, together with other exercises which I have shared with you, along with a series of stretching exercises.

Since, and during the Corona virus (COVID-19) pandemic, many thousands of employees from all over the world have been in lockdown and been forced working from home.

Mark Zuckerberg, Facebooks' chief executive, explained that they were looking at fully remote hiring to add employees away from its main offices in Silicon Valley and London.

He went on to add that half of its 45,000 staff will work from home, permanently and hinted at major home working innovations.

Colleagues would appear as realistic virtual characters and home workspaces would include 'floating screens' viewed through a virtual reality headset.

Guidelines for their Oculus headsets suggest a break every 30 minutes to prevent cyber sickness. Plus, an exercise regime. As more and more companies move to allow home working on a permanent basis their employees need to keep fit to work efficiently.

During and since the Corona virus (COVID-19) pandemic, many thousands of employees from all over the world have been in lockdown and been forced into working from home.

A physical therapist can give you invaluable advice to ease a back pain situation, along with other exercises, which I would like to share with you. Together with a *series of stretching exercises,* also what should be done to help ease the stiffness and pain.

Any of the exercises in my book can be used to relieve your sore back. Being static for too long is a major cause of aches and pains.

The fact that millions of us have been in lockdown due to the Corona virus working from home, and the speed that this has happened, has meant that home offices have been the order of the day.

Images have appeared on various social media of makeshift desks, kitchen tables, cocktail cabinets, stacks of boxes, etc. Certainly a recipe for back pain.

The Back Pain Survival Guide

The seven advisory tips to look after your back if you work from home are as follows.

- Move regularly. *Inactivity* is the biggest cause contributing factor in the rise of people suffering from back and neck pain and sciatica. Every twenty or thirty minutes stand up and move around.

- Climb the stairs or stretch to increase blood flow to the joints.

- When working on your computer make sure elbows are at 90 degrees

- If you are working from a laptop, raise your monitor up on some books so that the screen is at eye level.

- Avoid working away from your desk. On a sofa or bed for instance.

- Walk up and down the stairs if you are unable to access outside space.

- The final tip is to use an ironing board as a standing desk for variety. Being static for too long is a major recipe for disaster.

Chapter 11

Keeping Going

The Back Pain Survival Guide

Congratulations on making it this far in the book. Not only reading but doing the exercises I hope.

Remember, these are gentle stretching exercises, not part of a rigorous time trial workout. Do them and enjoy them. In return they will not only help ease back pain problems but also help you to avoid getting back pain.

Stretching is important. Rarely will you see a cat or dog rise from a long rest without doing their stretching routines. Make these exercises part of your daily routine.

You may find, as I did, one exercise in particular gives you the most benefit. I suggest you make that one a daily habit then add others to your routine over time. We all lapse our exercise periods at some time. Adding one exercise at a time helps to make them habit forming and much easier to keep going. The occasional miss is not a problem. Continually missing could be a problem.

Important... please be aware too of your posture daily. Bad posture can lead to problems you don't want.

Thank you for purchasing this book and allowing me to share my experiences with you. Wishing you all the best for the future.

Colin Platt

Chapter 12

Also Written by Colin Platt

Also written by Colin Platt

Healing Help from Honey Bees

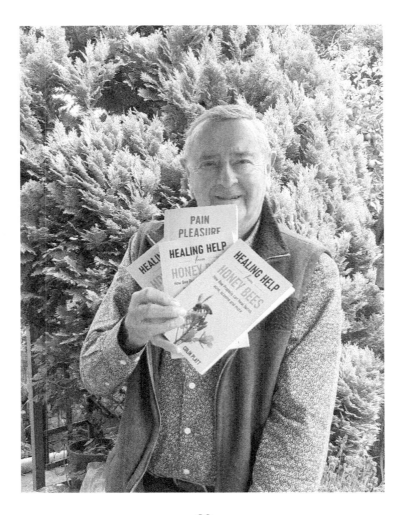

Also written by Colin Platt

I would appreciate if you would review my book on Amazon with the view to helping others with the solution to their back pain problems.

Finally, if I can help you further, please email me at: colinp07@gmail.com.

Chapter 13

Physical Therapy Association Offices

The Back Pain Survival Guide

American Physical Therapy Association

1111 North Fairfax Street
Alexandria
VA 22314
United States

www.apta.org

Australian Physiotherapy Association

Level 1, 1175 Toorak Road
Camberwell
Vic 3124
Australia

www.physiotherapy.asn.au

Argentine Association of Kinesiology

Virrey Liniers 1250
C1241ABB
Capital Federal
Argentina

www.aak.org.ar

Physiotherapists' Association of Brazil

Rua Carlos de Vasconcelos 111
Tijuca
Rio de Janeiro
Brazil

www.afb.org.br

Canadian Physiotherapy Association

955 Green Valley Crescent, Suite 270
Ottawa
ON K2C 3V4
Canada

www.physiotherapy.ca

Association of Danish Physiotherapists

Holmbladsgade 70
2300 Kobenhavn S
Denmark

www.fysio.dk

The Back Pain Survival Guide

French National Council of Physiotherapists

91 bis rue du Cherche Midi
75006 Paris
France

www.ordremk.fr/

German Association for Physiotherapy

Postfach 210280
Koln
D-50528
Germany

www.physio-deutschland.de

Italian Association of Physiotherapists

Via Pinerolo 3
Rome
00182
Italy

www.aifi.net

Japanese Physical Therapy Association

3-8-5 Sendagaya
Shibuya-ku
Tokyo
Japan

Mexican Association of Physiotherapy

Circ Interior Juan Pablo II # 1703 int 102
Col. Prados de agua azul
Puebla
Pue
Mexico

www.amefi.com.mx/

Royal Dutch Society for Physiotherapy

Stadsring 159b
P O Box 248
Amersfoort
3800 AE
Netherlands

www.kngf.nl

Physiotherapy New Zealand

P O Box 27 386
Marion Square
Wellington
614 New Zealand

pnz.org.nz/

Nigeria Society of Physiotherapy

c/o Physiotherapy Department
National Hospital
Abuja
Nigeria

www.nigeriaphysio.org

Spanish Association of Physiotherapists

Calle Conde de Penalver
Numero 38-2 dcha
28006 Madrid
Spain

www.aefi.net

Physical Therapy Association Offices

Chartered Society of Physiotherapy

14 Bedford Row
London
WC1R 4ED
United Kingdom

www.csp.org.uk

Index

A

Acupuncture · 8, 77, 80
Amazon · 89
Association Offices · 8, 91

B

Back Pain · 1, 3, 8, 14, 16, 38, 39, 40, 47, 62, 63, 73, 74, 76, 77, 82, 83, 89
Back Stretch · 7, 32, 33

C

Cat Camel · 7, 30, 31
Chiropractor · 8, 12, 74, 75
Cobra · 2, 3, 7, 34, 35, 36
Core · 7, 23, 25, 33, 37, 38, 39, 41, 42, 43, 45, 46, 47, 49, 57, 63
Corona virus · 82, 83
COVID-19 · 82, 83

D

Deportment · 8, 62, 63
Dynamic · 53

E

Extension, The Cobra · 7, 34, 35, 36

F

Frozen Shoulder · 69

G

Glutes · 25, 41, 46

H

Huggie · 7, 16, 28, 29, 71

I

Inclined push-ups · 50

L

Lifting · 8, 21, 39, 60, 61

The Back Pain Survival Guide

O

Obliques · 27
Oculus · 82
Osteopath · 8, 74, 76

P

Physical Therapy · 8, 74, 91, 92, 95
Physician · 12, 47, 55, 80
Posture · 7, 8, 16, 18, 20, 21, 24, 25, 34, 47, 62, 63, 64, 65, 74, 76, 86
Pregnancy · 7, 37, 38, 40
Prenatal · 7, 37, 40, 42
Push Ups · 8, 56, 57, 58

Q

Quadriceps · 53, 61

R

Rag Doll · 1, 2, 7, 15, 16, 22, 23
Reflexology · 8, 79, 80
Review · 6, 89

S

Sciatic Nerve · 8, 29, 70, 71
Shoulder · 8, 20, 23, 25, 27, 29, 31, 33, 35, 41, 42, 43, 47, 49, 50, 54, 55, 57, 58, 64, 65, 68, 69
Side Bend · 7, 26, 27
Spine · 27, 31, 46, 61, 63, 71, 75
Standing · 21, 23, 34, 36, 53, 84
Static · 53, 83, 84
Stretching · 1, 8, 15, 52, 53, 55, 58, 76, 82, 83

T

The Bridge · 7, 24, 25, 47
Tips · 8, 59, 71, 84
Training · 7, 14, 37, 42, 46, 47
Trimester · 7, 38, 39, 40, 41, 42, 43

W

Working From Home · 8, 81, 82, 83

Z

Zuckerberg, Mark · 82

Printed in Great Britain
by Amazon